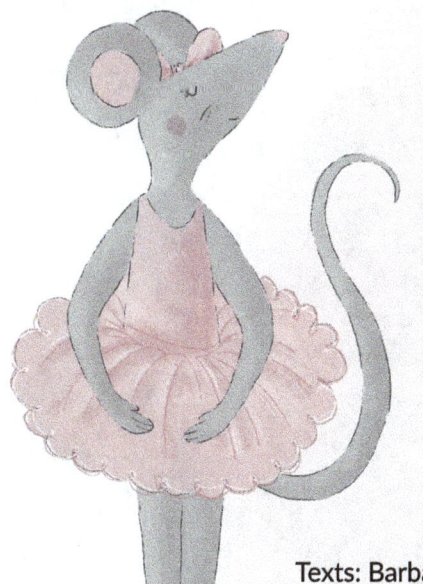

To my passion for dancing.

This book is dedicated to my students and to my two children, Sandrine and Antoine, the loves of my life.

Texts: Barbara Desrochers
Proofreading (of the French text): Marie-Josée Poulin
English Translation: Déborah Lafont
Illustrations: Marie Prévost
ISBN number: 978-1-387-40218-2

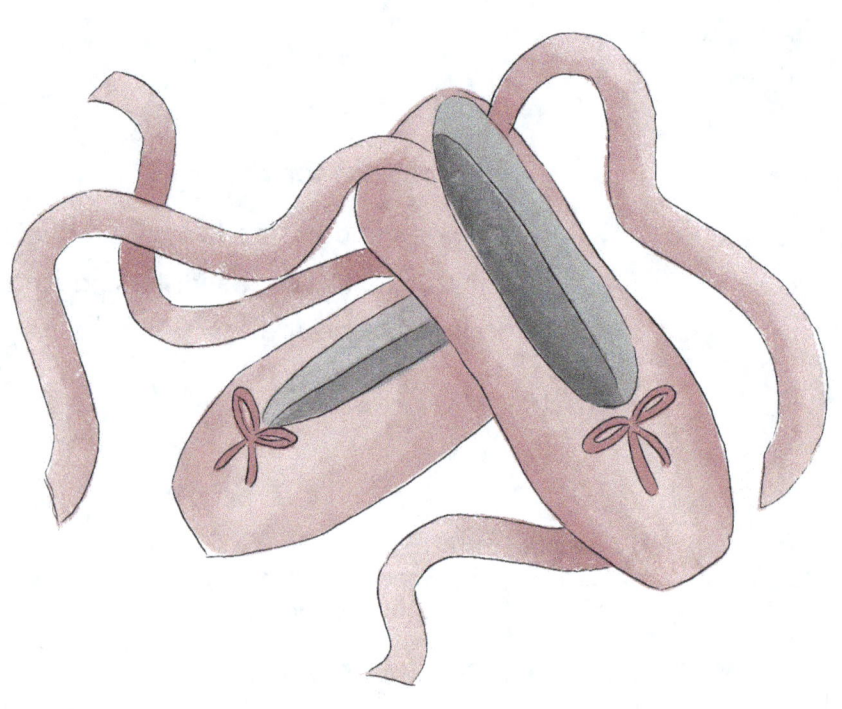

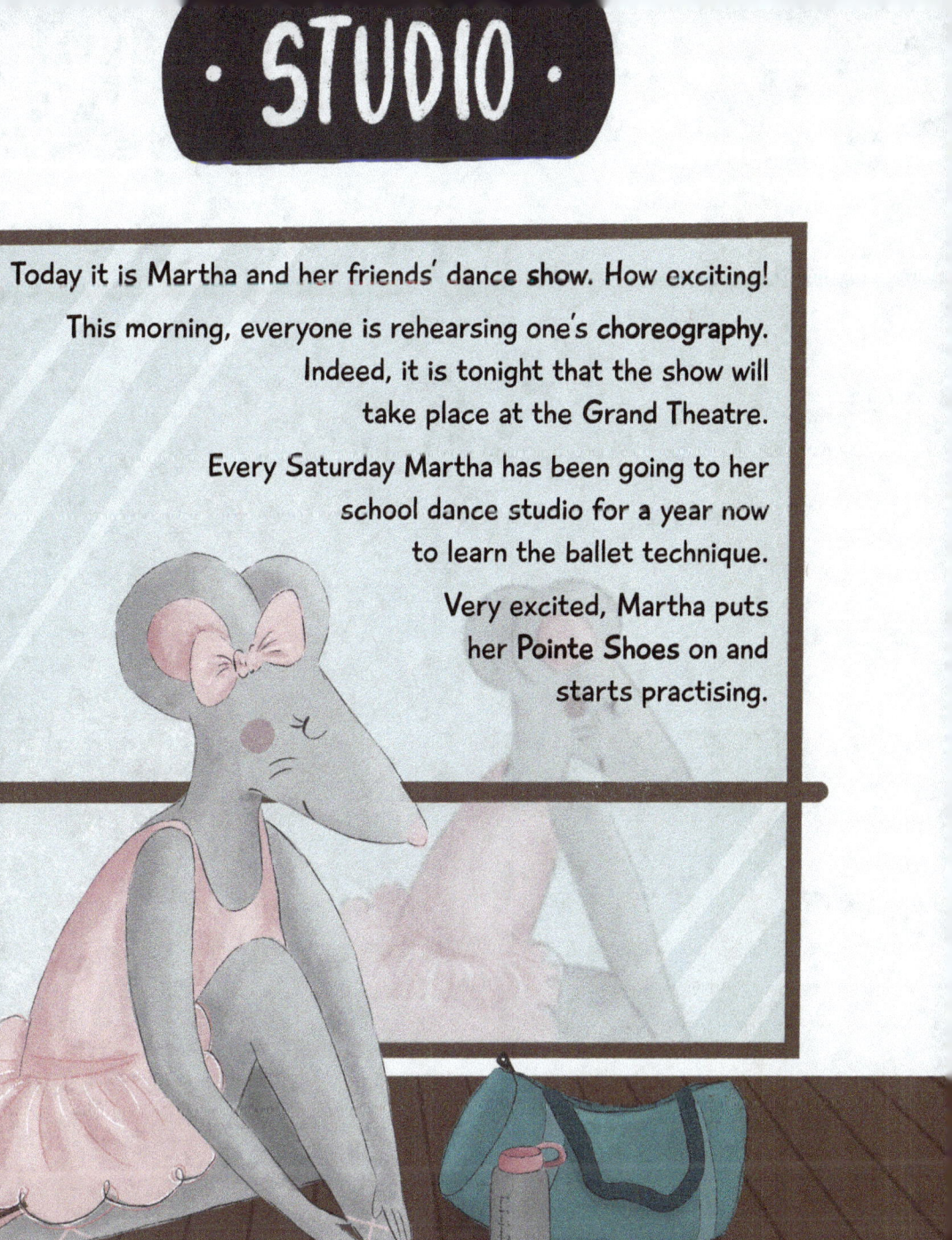

Today it is Martha and her friends' dance show. How exciting!

This morning, everyone is rehearsing one's **choreography**. Indeed, it is tonight that the show will take place at the Grand Theatre.

Every Saturday Martha has been going to her school dance studio for a year now to learn the ballet technique.

Very excited, Martha puts her **Pointe Shoes** on and starts practising.

-3-

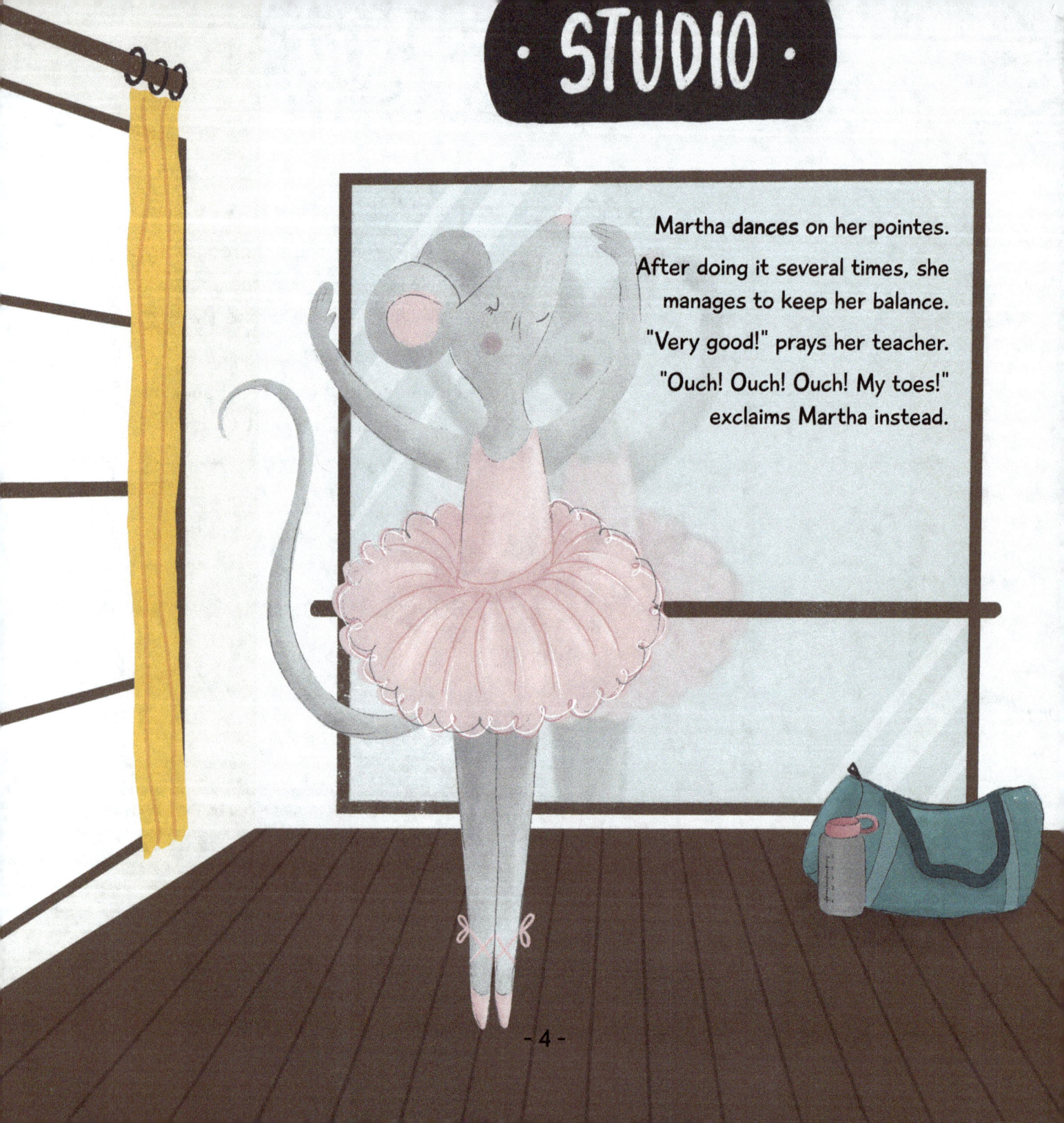

STUDIO

Martha **dances** on her pointes.
After doing it several times, she
manages to keep her balance.
"Very good!" prays her teacher.
"Ouch! Ouch! Ouch! My toes!"
exclaims Martha instead.

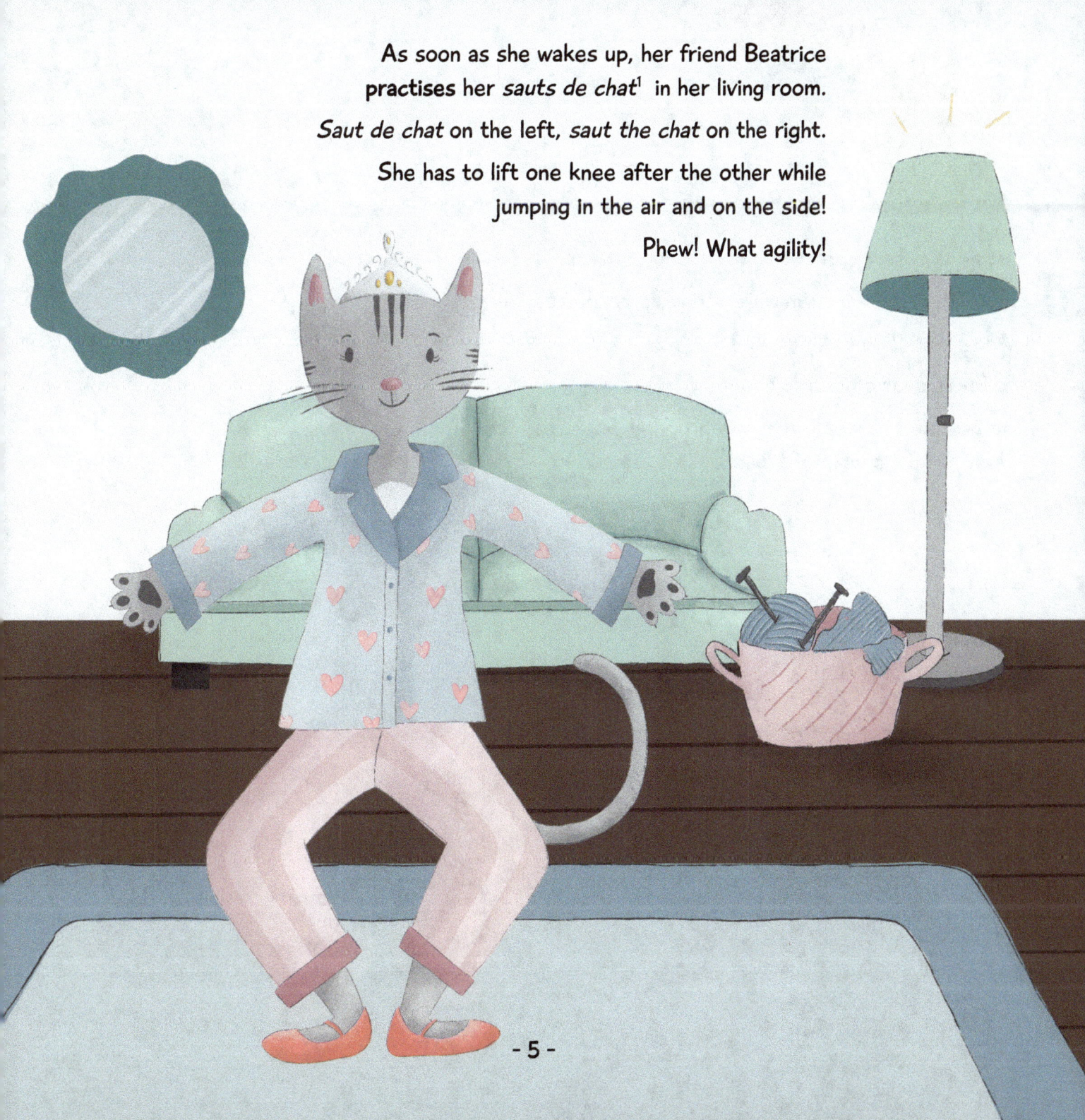

As soon as she wakes up, her friend Beatrice **practises** her *sauts de chat*[1] in her living room.

Saut de chat on the left, *saut the chat* on the right.

She has to lift one knee after the other while jumping in the air and on the side!

Phew! What agility!

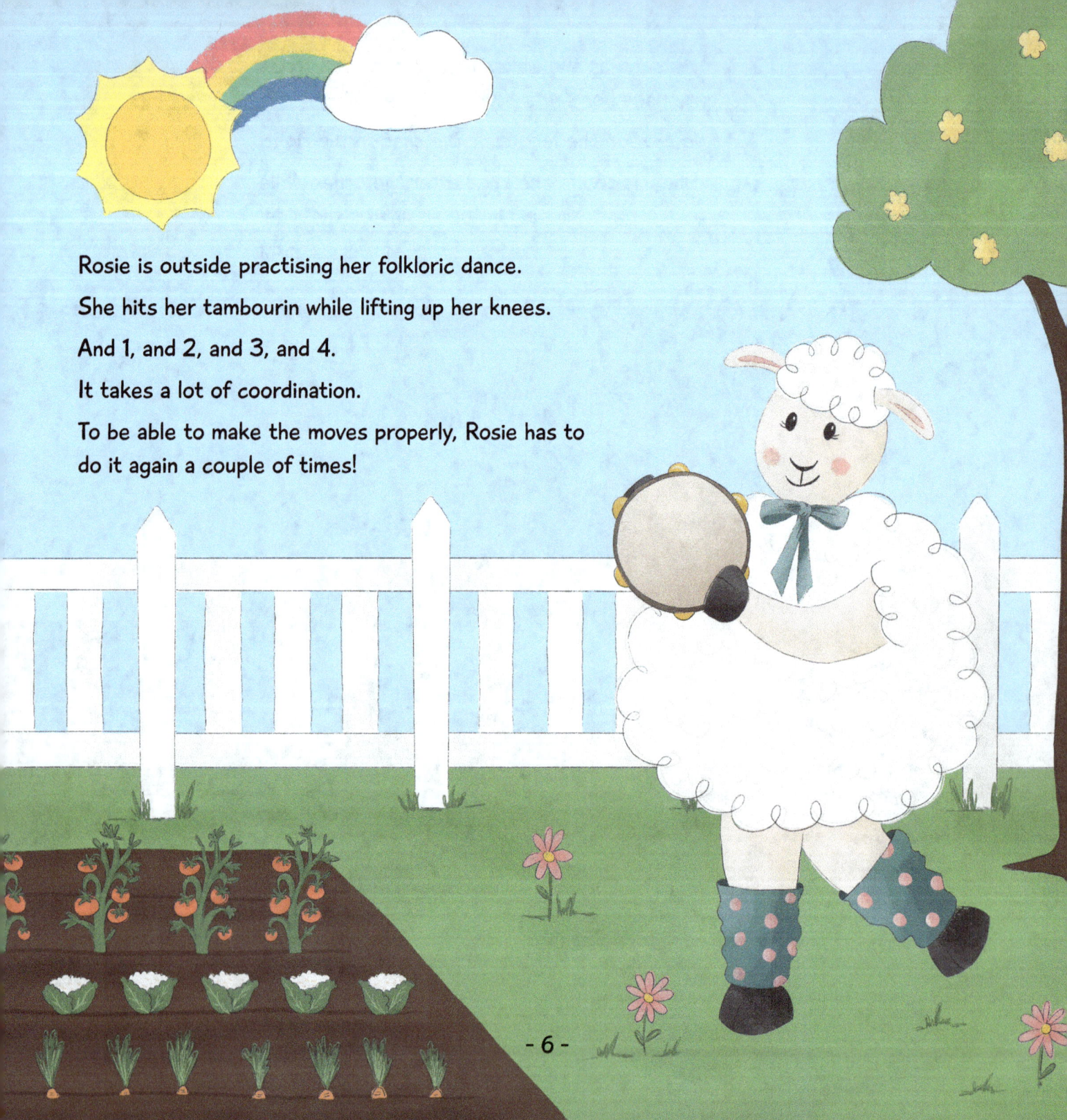

Rosie is outside practising her folkloric dance.

She hits her tambourin while lifting up her knees.

And 1, and 2, and 3, and 4.

It takes a lot of coordination.

To be able to make the moves properly, Rosie has to do it again a couple of times!

This is Hubert. He is gambolling to the studio for the **rehearsal**.

He is a bit late!

Two steps forward and one step back. Hip hop!

He would not want to make a mistake when the curtain goes up, because his whole family will be there tonight for the show!

He is keeping up the rhythm.

"Hurry up, Hubert!"

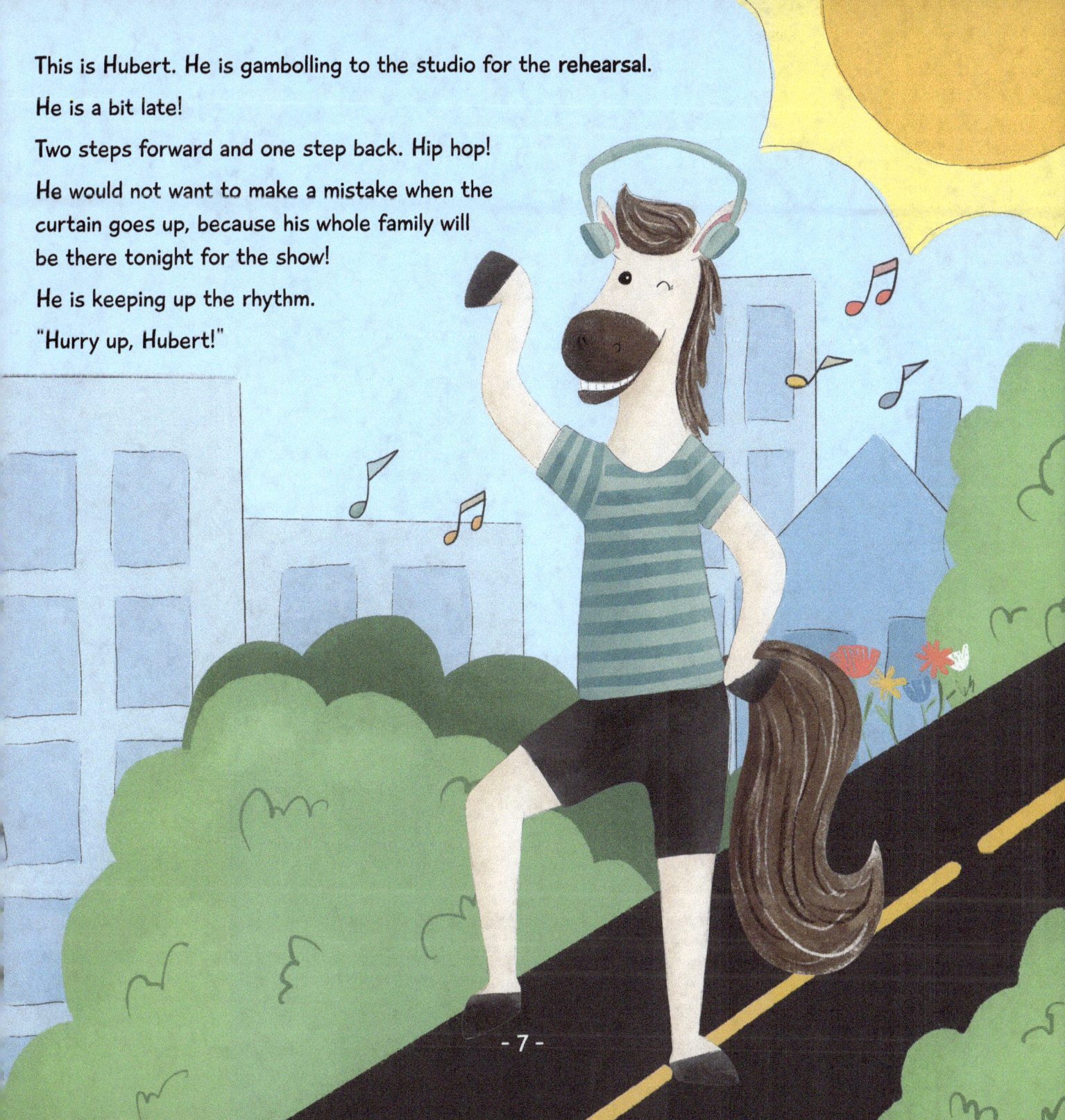

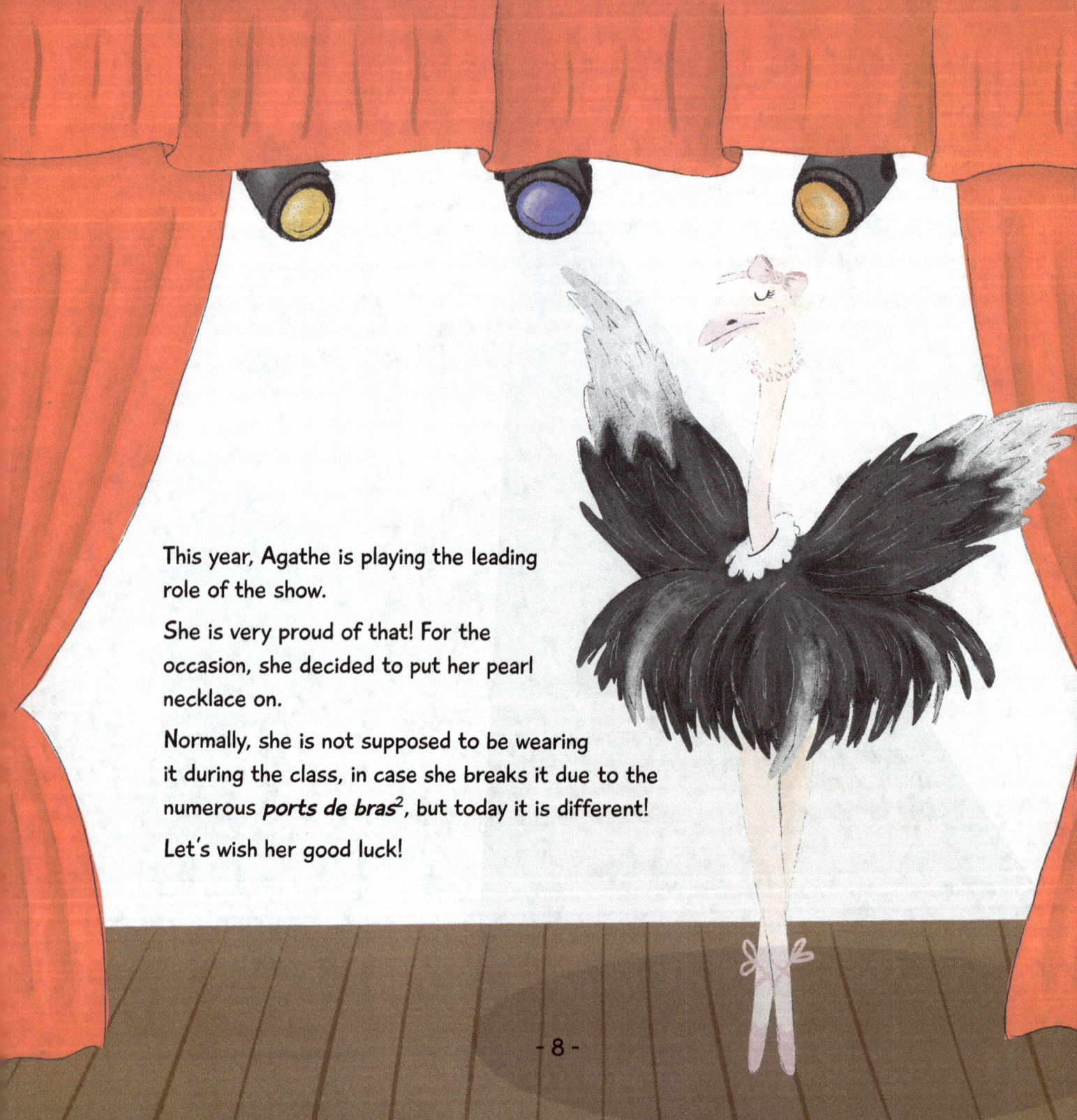

This year, Agathe is playing the leading role of the show.

She is very proud of that! For the occasion, she decided to put her pearl necklace on.

Normally, she is not supposed to be wearing it during the class, in case she breaks it due to the numerous *ports de bras*[2], but today it is different!

Let's wish her good luck!

The triplets, Fanny, Flore and Fiona, will be part of the *corps de ballet*[3].
Arabesques, *pirouettes*[4], *fouettés*[5], and *cabrioles*[6]. They are so graceful!
Well done, ladies! How pretty you are with your magnificent *tutus*[7]!

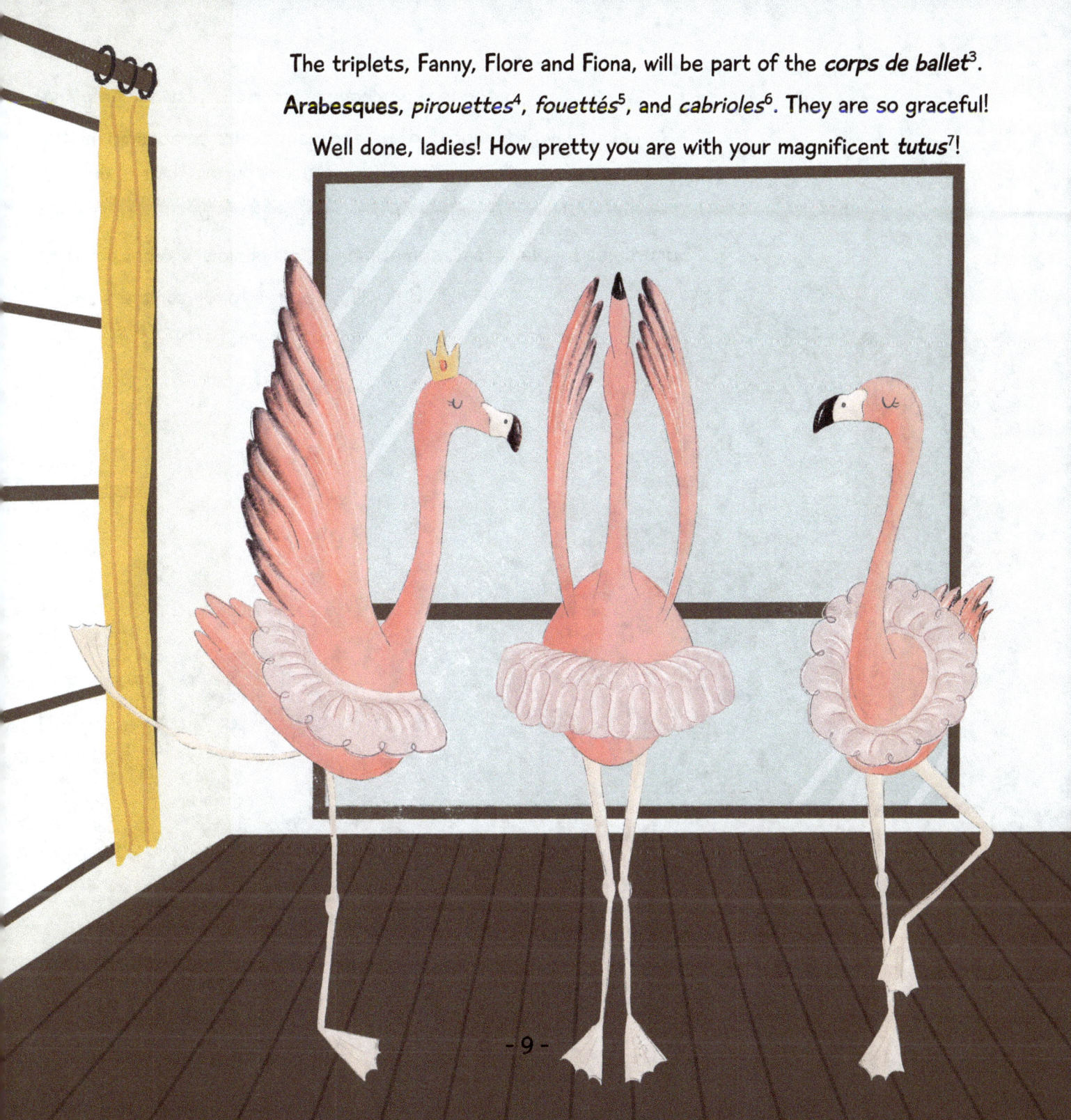

Leon is the accompanist. He is playing the piano.

He could play different rhythms for many hours to accompany the dancers during their exercises.

A waltz here, an adagio there or else an **allegro**.

Sometimes he plays fast, sometimes he plays slowly. What a talent!

But will he be ready for tonight's show?

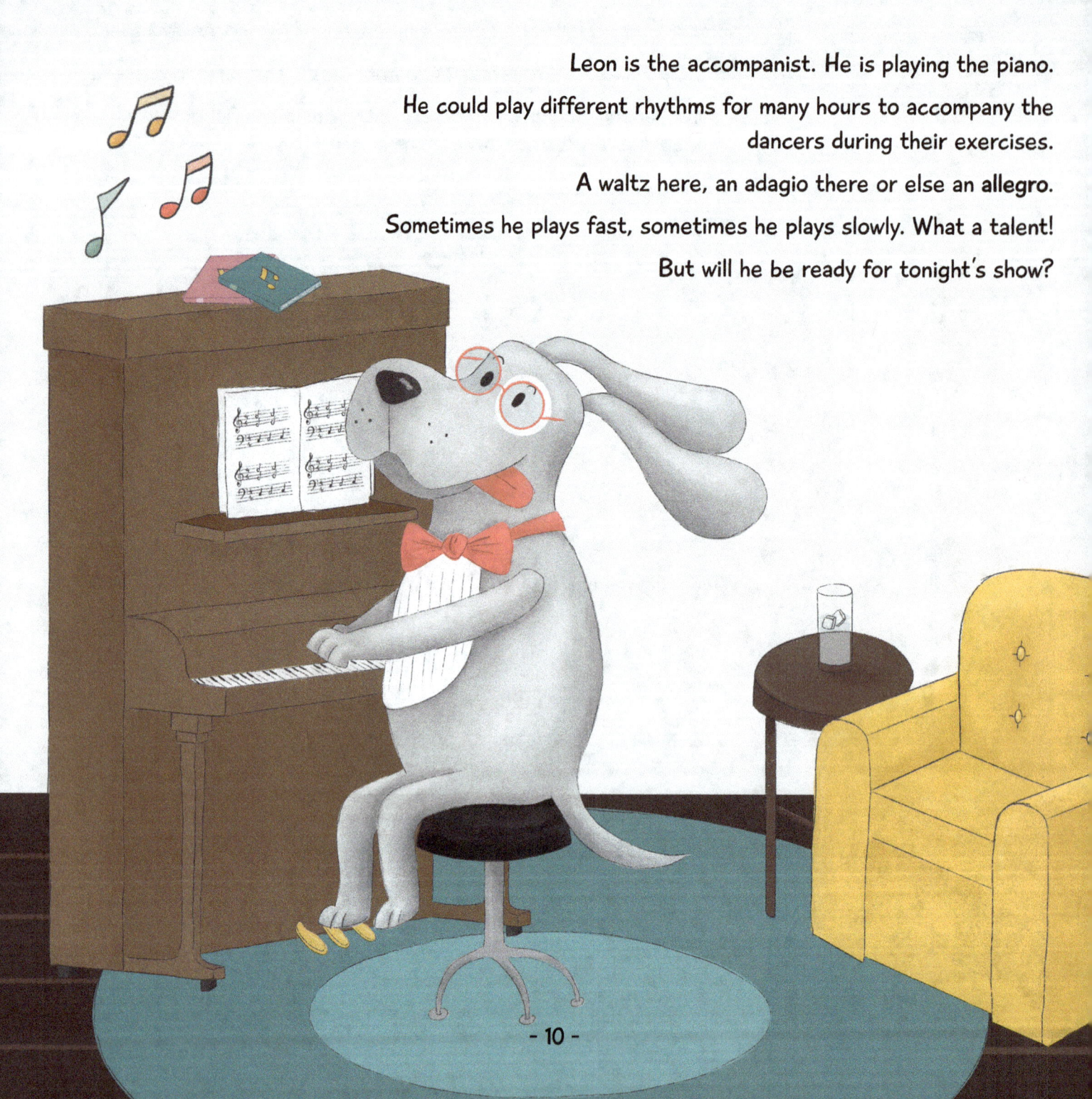

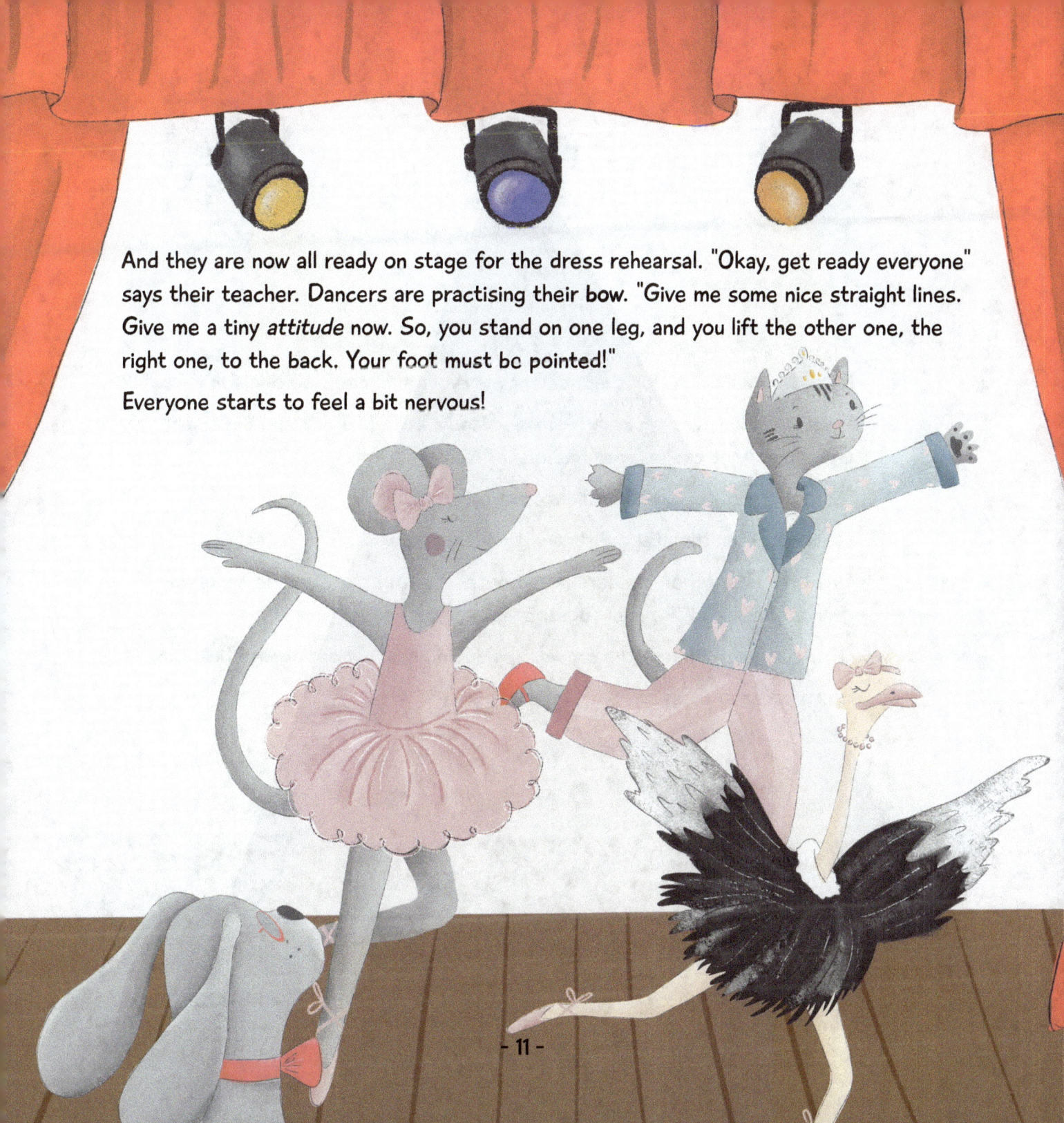

And they are now all ready on stage for the dress rehearsal. "Okay, get ready everyone" says their teacher. Dancers are practising their bow. "Give me some nice straight lines. Give me a tiny *attitude* now. So, you stand on one leg, and you lift the other one, the right one, to the back. Your foot must be pointed!"

Everyone starts to feel a bit nervous!

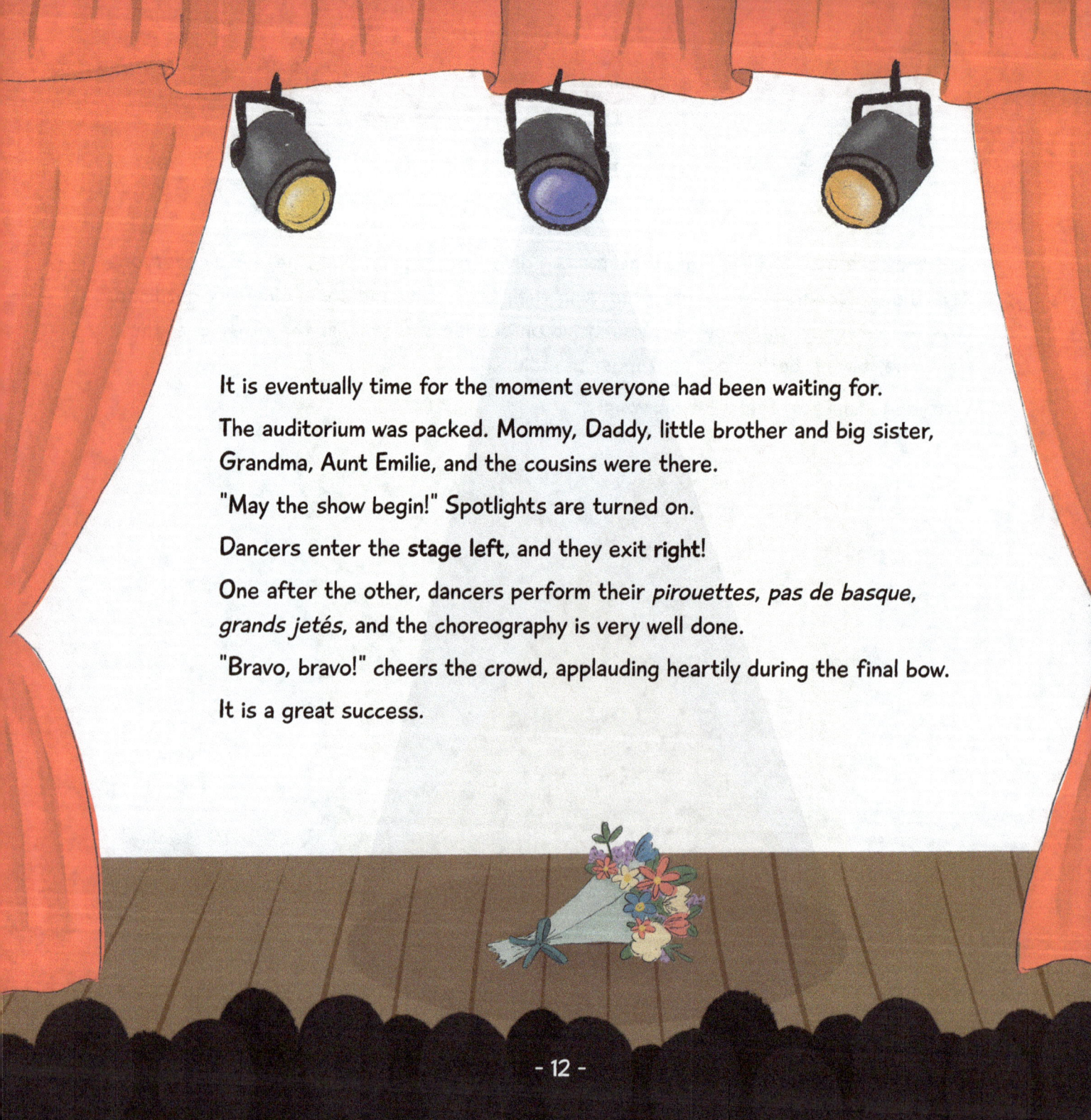

It is eventually time for the moment everyone had been waiting for.

The auditorium was packed. Mommy, Daddy, little brother and big sister, Grandma, Aunt Emilie, and the cousins were there.

"May the show begin!" Spotlights are turned on.

Dancers enter the **stage left**, and they exit **right**!

One after the other, dancers perform their *pirouettes, pas de basque, grands jetés,* and the choreography is very well done.

"Bravo, bravo!" cheers the crowd, applauding heartily during the final bow.

It is a great success.

The show was so fabulous that no one realized that Martha did not manage to keep her balance on her pointes,

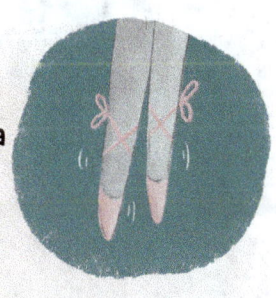

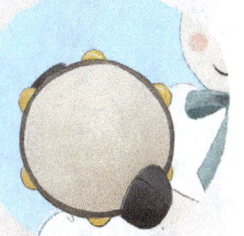

that Beatrice hurt her toe landing on
the floor after her *saut de chat*,

that Rosie hit her tambourin a bit too hard.

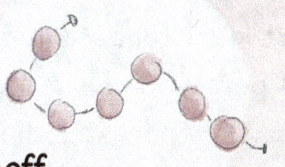

No one noticed that Hubert did three steps
forward rather than two,

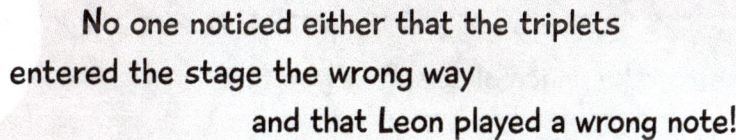

and that Agathe's necklace came off.

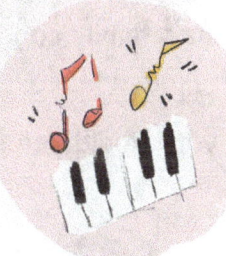

No one noticed either that the triplets
entered the stage the wrong way
and that Leon played a wrong note!

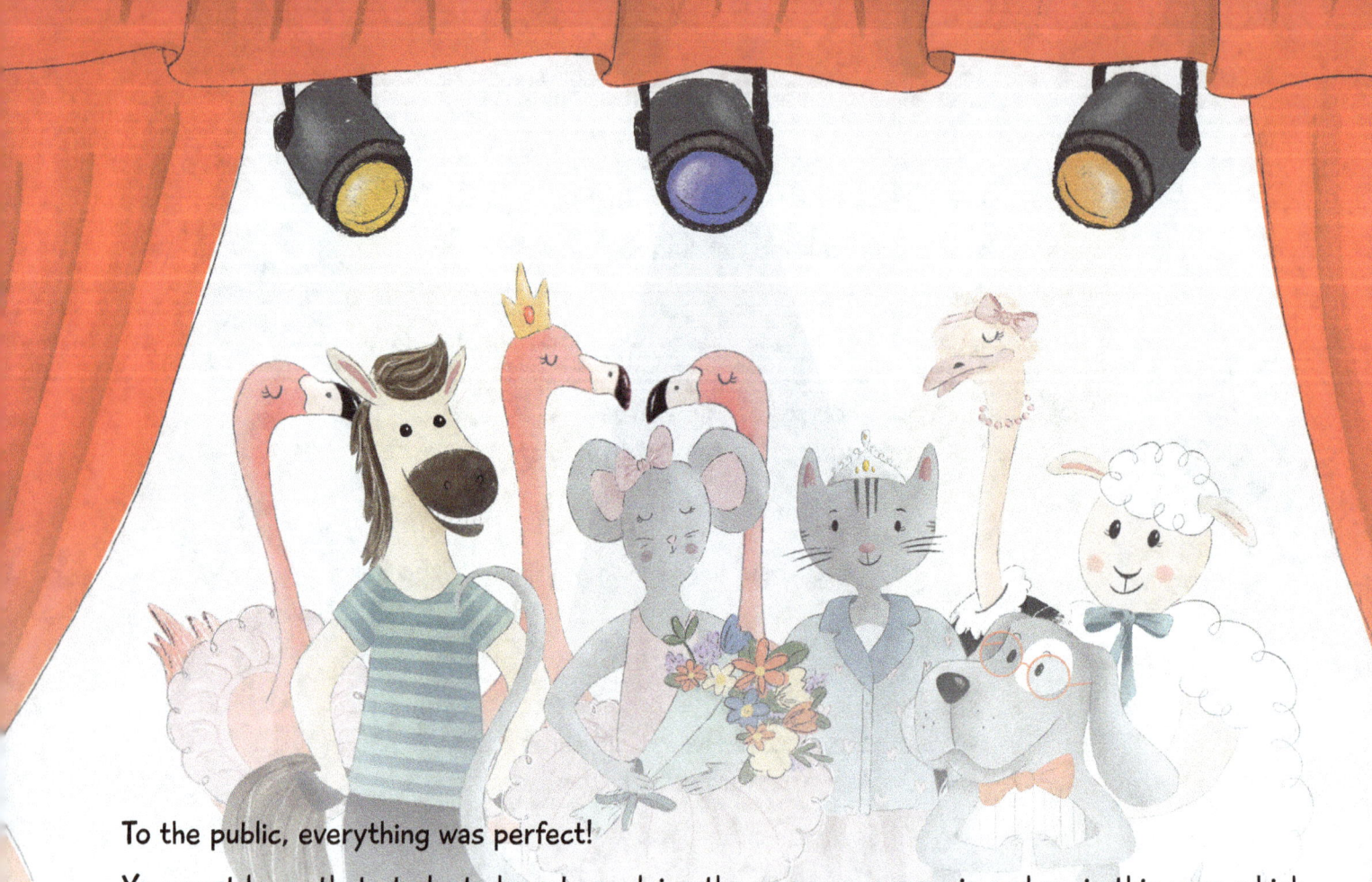

To the public, everything was perfect!

You must know that students have been doing the same moves again and again this year, which requires perseverance. Also, they made considerable effort and they put a lot of energy into their practice to master the technique and make a success of this show. Today, they are very proud and happy with the result, which just goes to show that one should never give up though one is faced with difficulties!

Martha's family congratulated her with a lovely bunch of flowers.
She enjoyed her experience so much that she is planning on doing it again next year.

And you, would you like to take dance classes?

Dance activities

Here are some exercises that you can do at home with Martha and her friends.

Choose your favourite music, and Bob's your uncle!

You do not have any? Here is what I suggest:
https://open.spotify.com/playlist/2xCje52JG7U3FIOXaePRMB.

The number of the playlist to use is indicated by the symbol #.

Enjoy!

*Practise the five ballet technical positions
with Martha, the mouse** #1

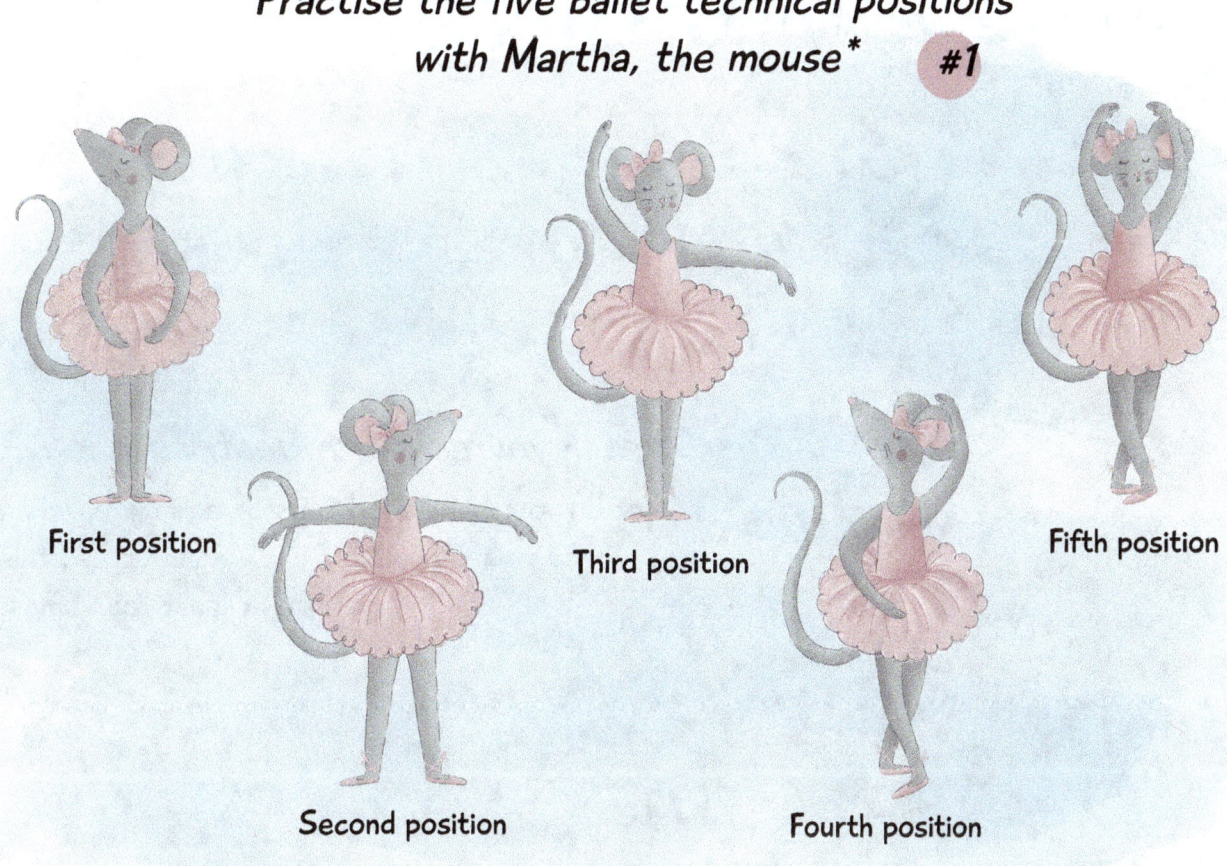

First position

Second position

Third position

Fourth position

Fifth position

* The position of the arms may vary according to the ballet technique used or to the country.

Strengthen your feet and ankles with Agathe, the ostrich

While standing, with the back well straight, walk on your demi-pointes. You can turn right, then left, and even have a break!

Do it over and over again if you like. I suggest that you put your hands on your waist; it will help!

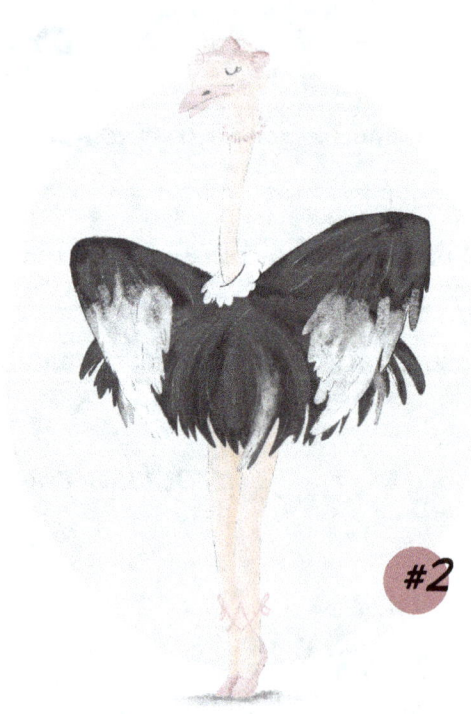

#2

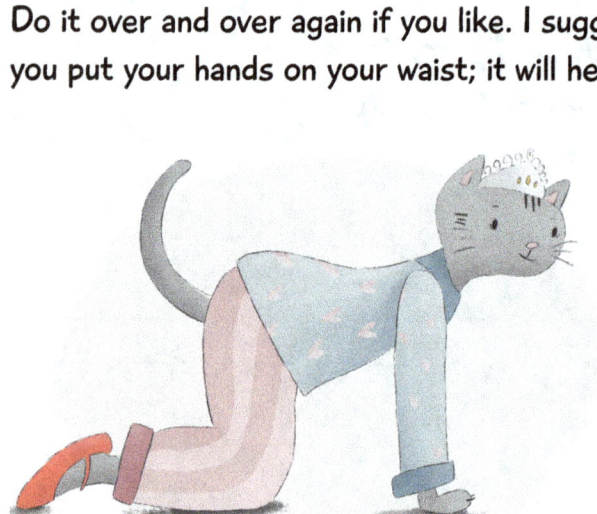

Stretch yourself with Beatrice, the cat

Get on your hand and knees on a flat area, then bend your back like a cat waking up. Do this exercise at least four times.

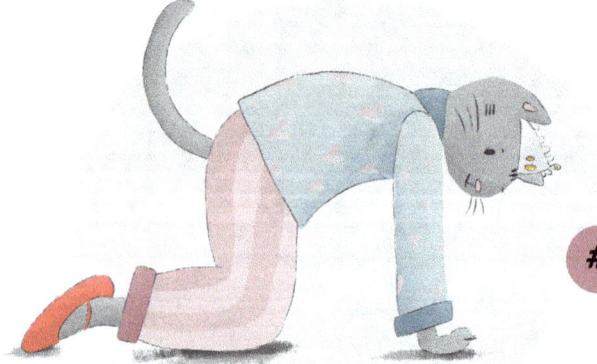

#3

The flamingo triplets

Keep your balance with Fanny

Stand on one leg, try and keep your balance for eight seconds. Then, try with the other leg.

Become suppler with Fiona

While standing, bend over to your feet and try to touch your toes. Take it easy!

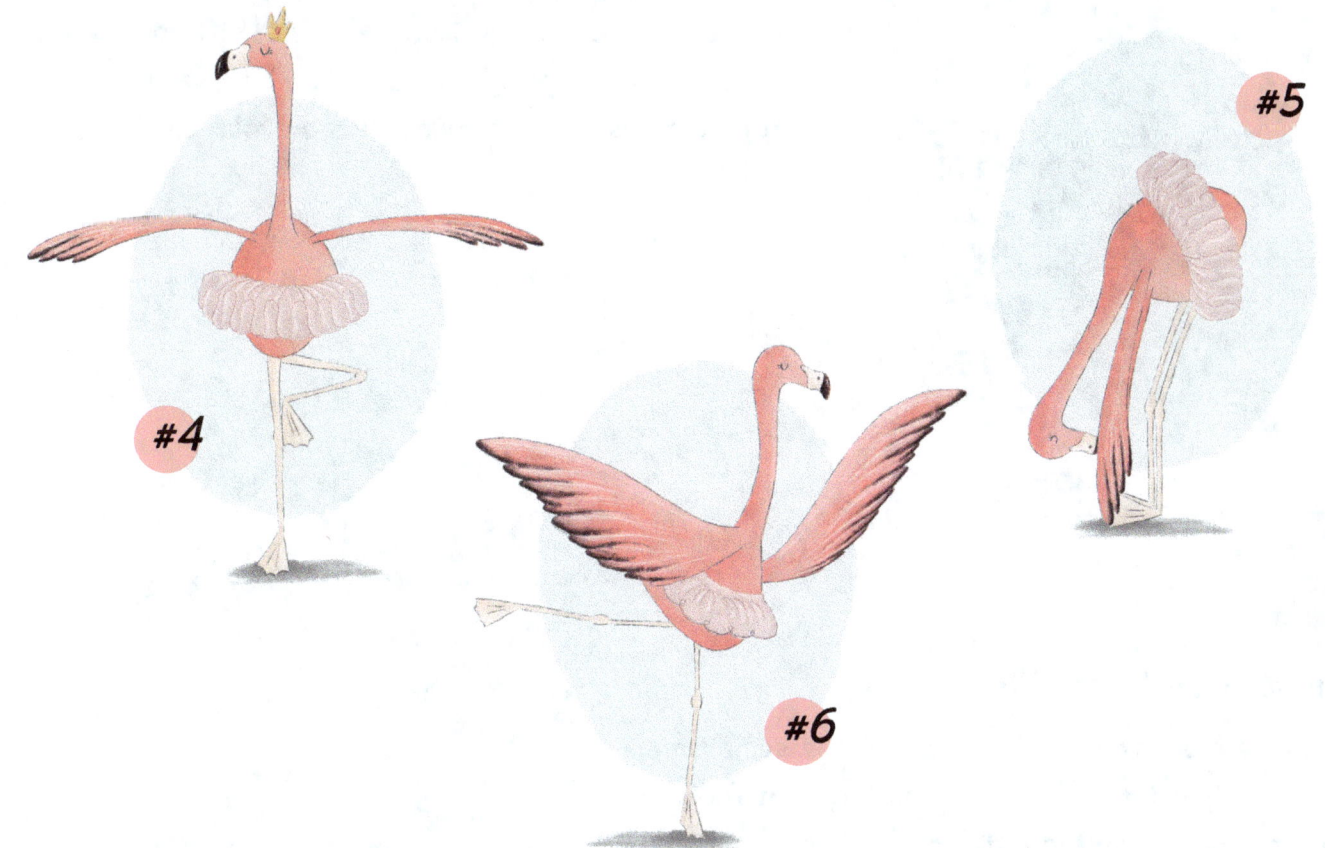

With Flore, do an arabesque for the first time

Extend one leg directly behind you. Place an arm on the side, and another one in front of you, just like Flore. This is a first arabesque!

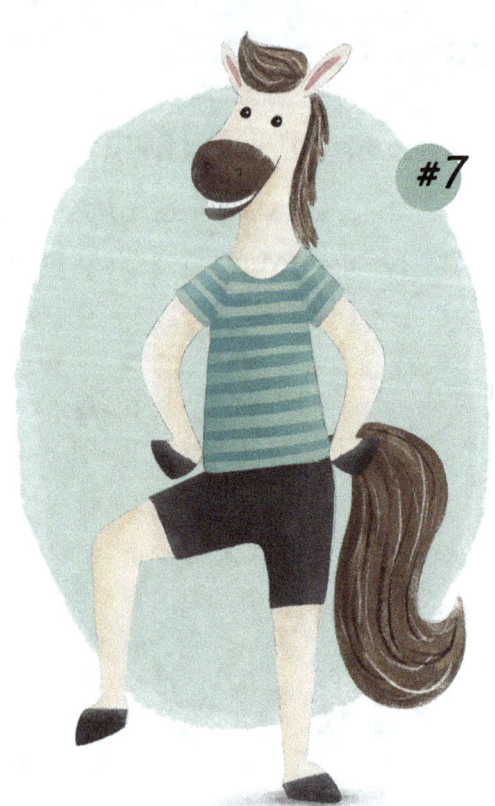

#7

Gambol with Hubert, the horse

Jump around your favourite teddy bear! Lift your knees while going forward, then backwards. You might as well put your hands on your waist.

Jump with Leon, the dog

Hop like a bunny, using both feet at the same time. Do this eight times. Then, hop on the right foot four times, and on the left foot four times. After this, repeat the exercise clapping your hands.

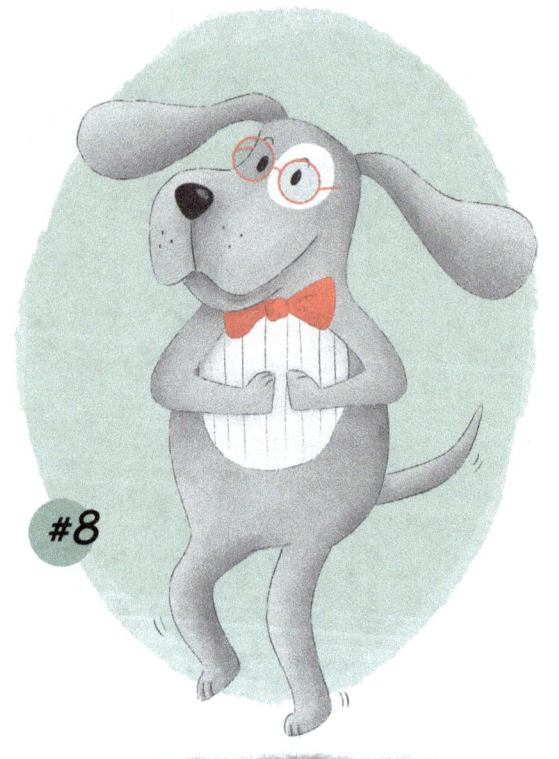

#8

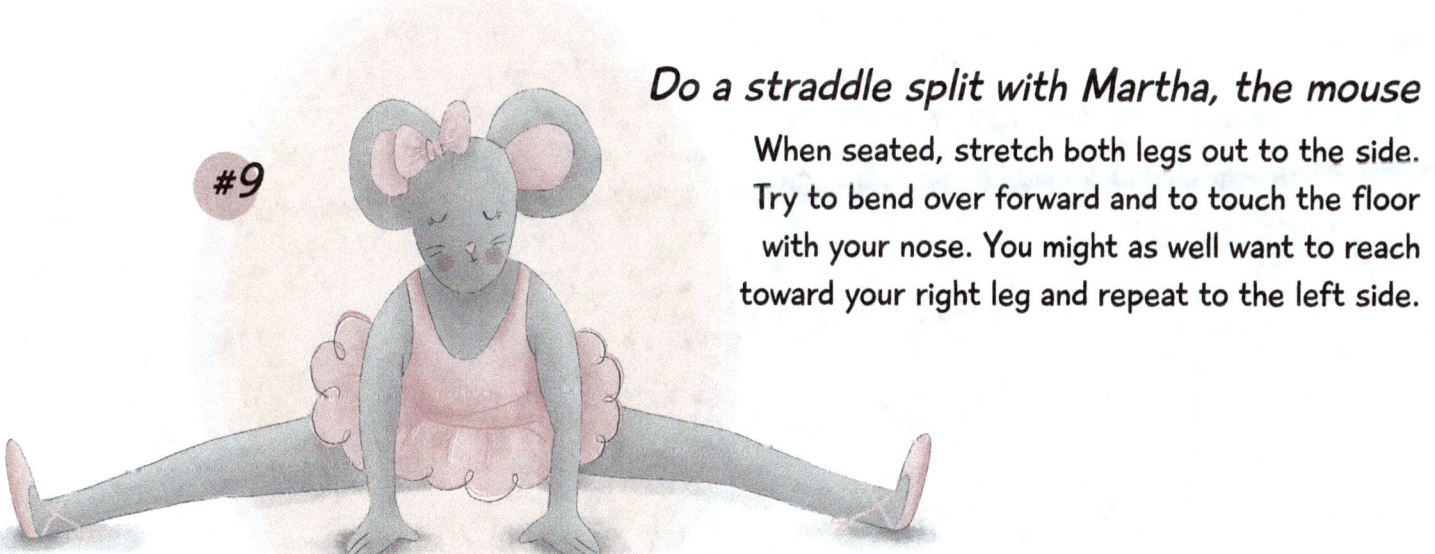

Do a straddle split with Martha, the mouse

#9

When seated, stretch both legs out to the side. Try to bend over forward and to touch the floor with your nose. You might as well want to reach toward your right leg and repeat to the left side.

Relax with Rosie, the sheep

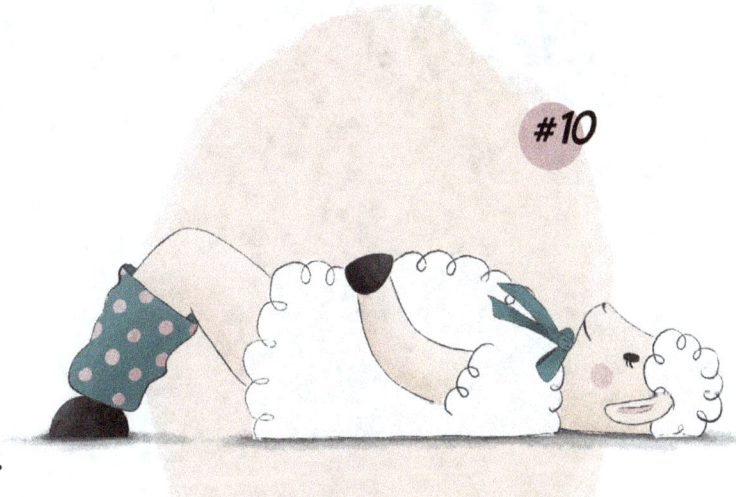

#10

Lay down on your back, bend your knees. Place your hands on your tummy. **INHALE** through your nose blowing your belly, then **EXHALE** through your mouth. You will notice your belly "deflate" as it gets empty. Repeat the exercise to ensure relaxation.

With your friends you can also dance a round!

Dance clockwise, then anticlockwise.

Then, gather in the middle and start again!

LET'S DANCE!

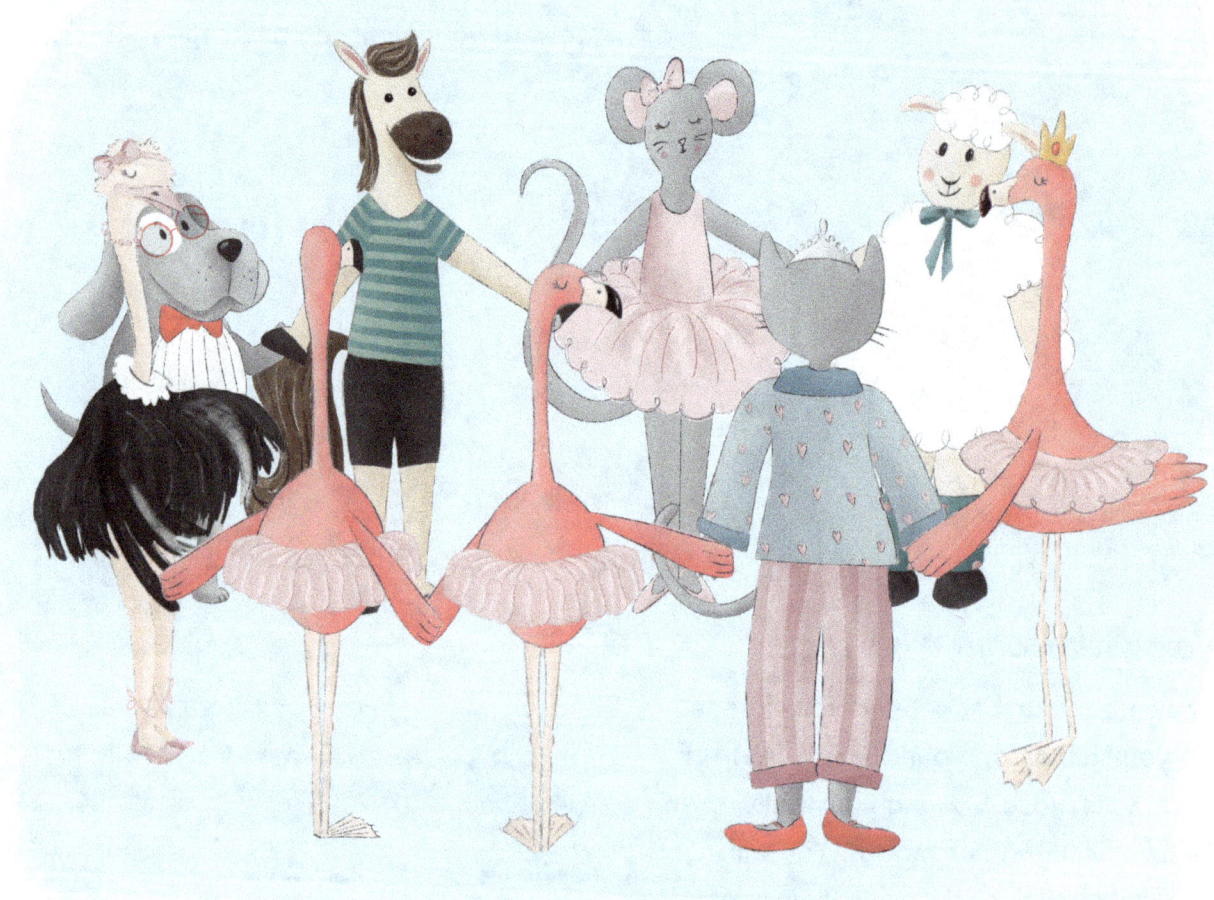

Now, I encourage you to make up your own exercises or choreography.

Get your creativity and imagination running!

You can use accessories like a hat, a scarf, a hoop, and put on a costume of your choice.

Have fun!

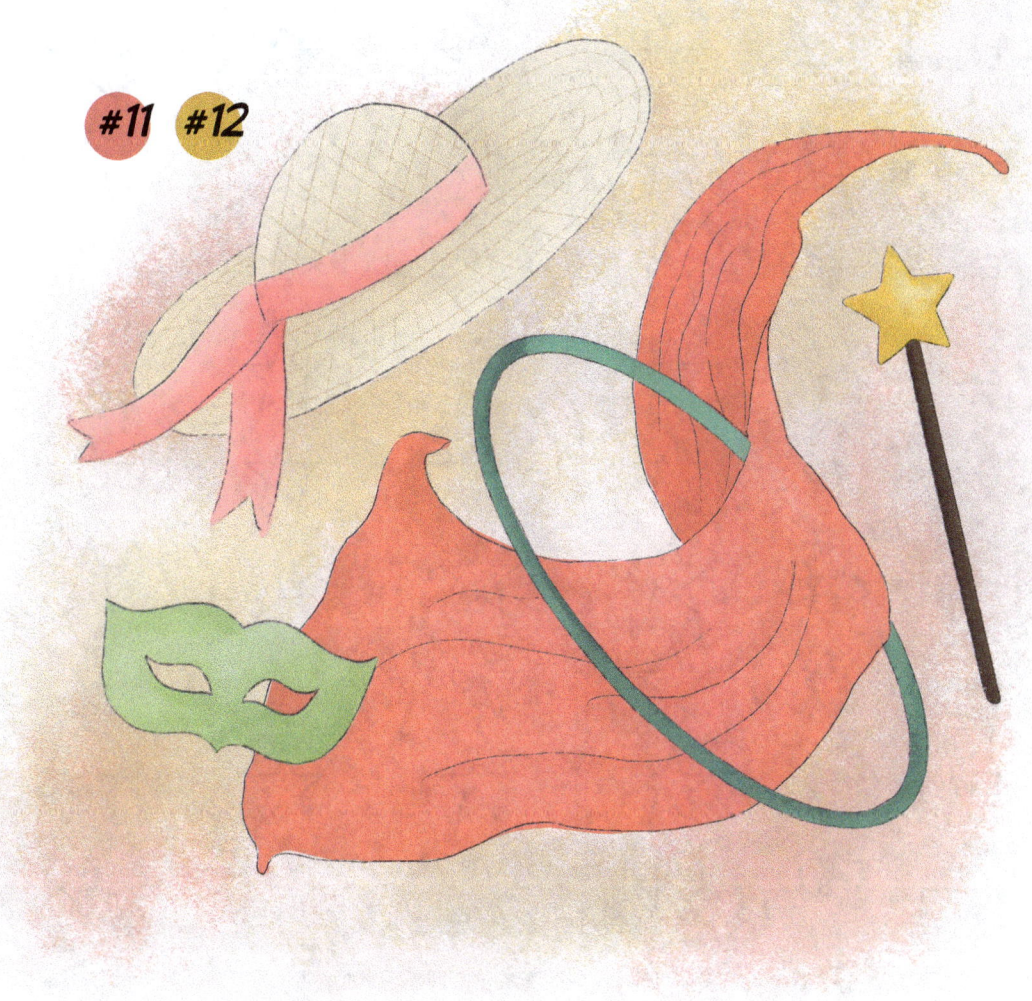

I did it!

Colour the stars according to your level of success. Be honest with yourself!

	Well	Very well	Great	Excellent	Congrats, you're a star!
Exercise #1	☆	☆	☆	☆	☆
Exercise #2	☆	☆	☆	☆	☆
Exercise #3	☆	☆	☆	☆	☆
Exercise #4	☆	☆	☆	☆	☆
Exercise #5	☆	☆	☆	☆	☆
Exercise #6	☆	☆	☆	☆	☆
Exercise #7	☆	☆	☆	☆	☆
Exercise #8	☆	☆	☆	☆	☆
Exercise #9	☆	☆	☆	☆	☆
Exercise #10	☆	☆	☆	☆	☆

Here are some ideas of snacks you could eat after exercising

☐ Fresh fruit (slices of apple, banana, pear, grapes, melon)

☐ Cheese cubes or sticks

☐ Yogurt pot or drink

☐ Raw veggies (carrots, celery, broccoli) (according to the child's age)

☐ Granola bar (not too sweet)

☐ Homemade muffin

☐ Rice cakes

☐ Water (enables the body to stay hydrated after exercising)

Ideally, it is recommended to offer the snack at least 2 hours prior to the next meal, so as not to spoil the lunch or dinner.

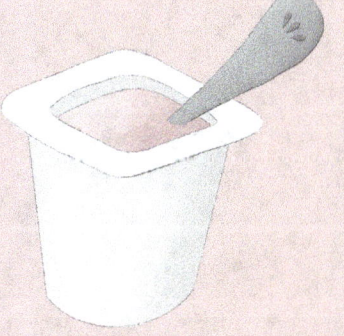

What to pack in your dance bag?

☐ Dance outfit

☐ Stockings

☐ Ballet skirt

☐ Ballet shoes (Pointe Shoes)

☐ Dance shoes for other dance styles

☐ Hairbrush

☐ Hairband

☐ Bobby pins for bun

☐ Hair nets for bun if necessary

☐ Water bottle

☐ A little snack to have after your class

☐ No jewelry, no gums

☐ Put a lovely smile on you face!

Have a great class!

Colouring pictures

Download the 7 colouring pictures of Martha and her friends on the website
of *Académie de danse Barbara Desrochers*, under the tab "MARTHA AIME LA DANSE".

https://www.ecolededansebarbara.com/

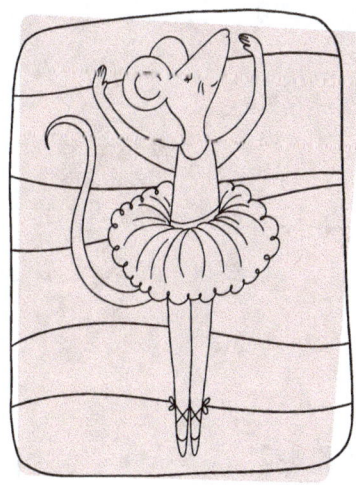 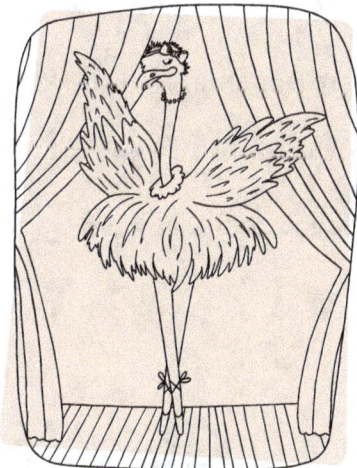 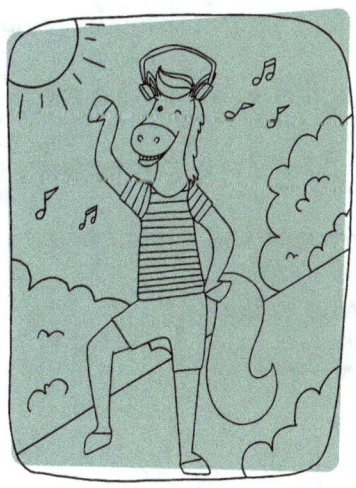

- If you have the opportunity, go and attend these famous ballets at least once in your life:

    - Swan Lake
    - The Nutcracker
    - Sleeping Beauty
    - *Coppélia*
    - *Giselle*

    - *La Bayadère*
    - Raymonda
    - Romeo & Juliet
    - *La Sylphide*
    - The Rite of Spring

Memory activities
For the answers, go to page 30.

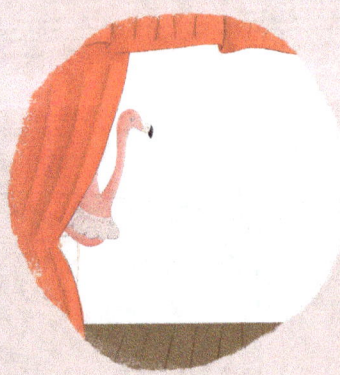

1. What does Martha have on her feet?

2. What is Beatrice practising?

3. Rosie is practising her dance...

4. Hubert is doing two steps forward and one...

5. Who will play the leading role of the show this year?

6. What is the name of the magnificent costume worn by the triplets?

7. Who is Leon?

To go further
For the answers, go to page 30.

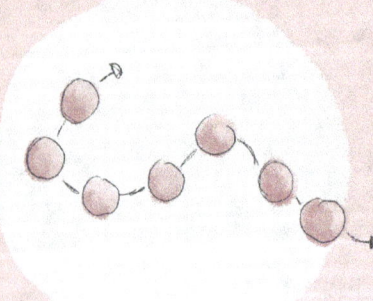

8. What are the triplets' names?

9. Name at least two dance steps performed by the triplets.

10. Which dance style does Hubert like?

11. What fall off Agathe's neck?

12. Where did Beatrice hurt herself?

13. What is the name of Rosie's percussion instrument?

14. By whom are the dancers applauded?

Hunt & Seek

Find the following items on the different pages of the book.
You will find the answers on page 30.

☐ A ballet barre

☐ Carrots

☐ A mirror

☐ Red shoes

☐ Pointe Shoes

☐ Music scores

☐ A tambourin

☐ A couch

☐ A tutu

☐ A golden crown

☐ A rainbow

☐ Cauliflowers

☐ A glass of water

☐ An arabesque leg

☐ A pearl necklace

☐ A piano

☐ A ball of wool

☐ A headset

☐ A bunch of flowers

☐ A striped T-shirt

Labyrinth

Help Martha find her Pointe Shoes again.
The answer will be on page 30.

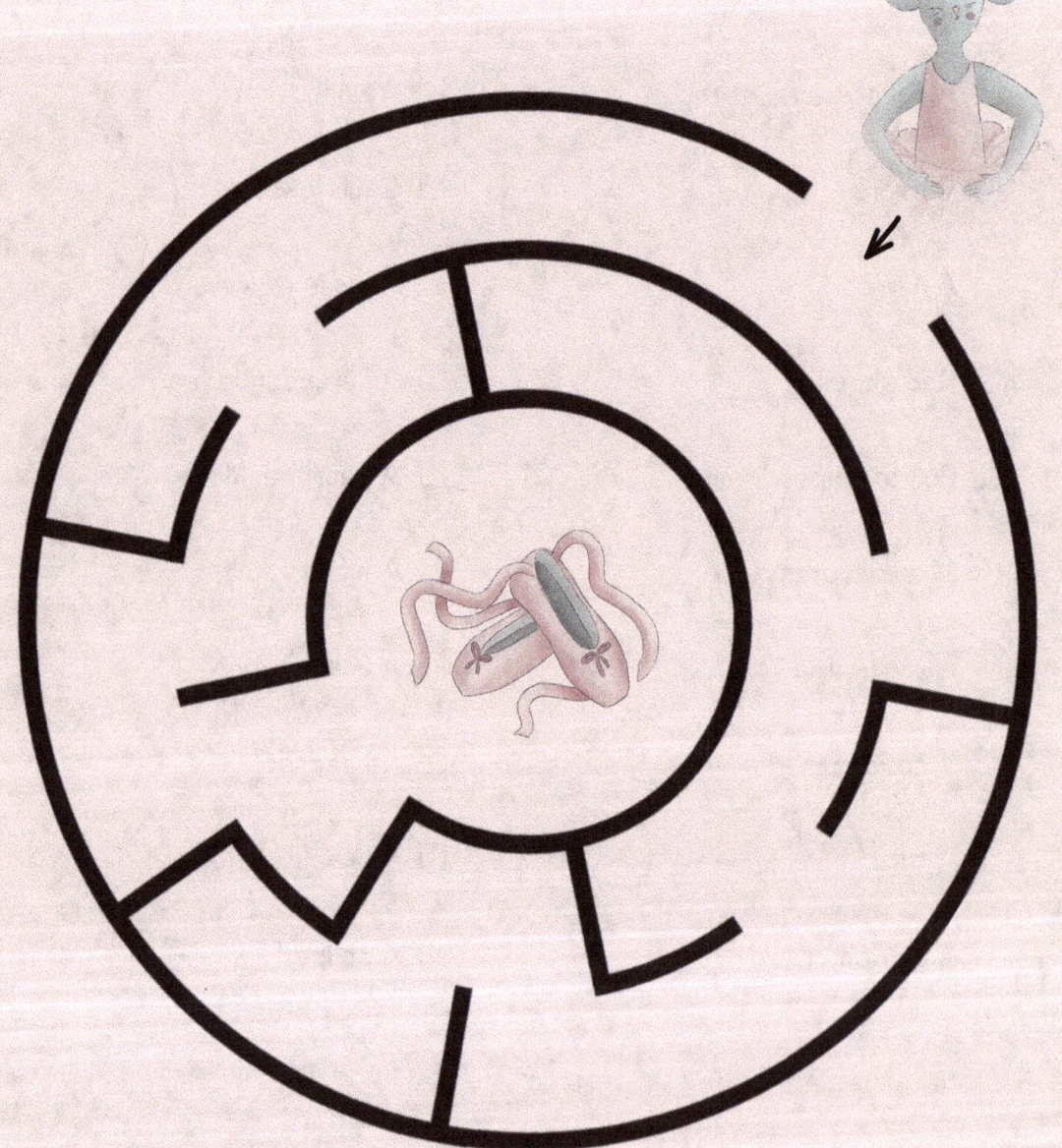

Vocabulary
(In the order of appearance in the text)

Show: an activity/performance which is done in front of a public.

Choreography: a series of dance steps that make up a ballet or dance.

Pointe Shoes: the shoes that ballerinas wear to be safely supported and dance on the tips of their toes in classical and contemporary ballet.

Dance: a pattern of movements that you make with your feet and your body, following the sound of music.

Rehearsal: occasions when you make the choreography moves or steps again and again before a show, in order to become better at it.

Port de bras: French word for "movement of the arms." It describes how dancers move their arms from one position to another.

Corps de ballet: refers to the dancers in a ballet that dance as a group.

Arabesque: a position in ballet dancing in which you lift one leg behind you, and that requires a sense of balance.

Tutu: a short skirt made of multiple tulle layers that a female classical ballet dancer usually wears.

Allegro: a piece of music that should be played or sung quickly.

Bow: the action of curtsying, bending forward from waist or bending knees with one leg behind the other.

Stage left: "Côté cour" in French. On the left side of the stage for a dancer who is looking towards the audience.

Stage right: "Côté jardin" in French. On the right side of the stage for an actor who is looking towards the audience.

These definitions were inspired and adapted for this children's book.
https://ballethub.com/ballet-terms-dictionary/
https://www.macmillandictionary.com/

Answers

Memory activities

1. Pointe Shoes
2. Sauts de chat
3. Folkloric
4. Back
5. Agathe
6. A tutu
7. The pianist or the accompanist

To go further

8. Flore, Fiona & Fanny
9. Arabesque, pirouette, fouetté & cabriole
10. Hip hop
11. Her pearl necklace
12. Her toe
13. A tambourin
14. The public, family & friends

Hunt & Seek

Page 3, 4, 9: a ballet barre, a mirror, Pointe Shoes

Page 5: a ball of wool, red ballet shoes, a couch

Page 6: a tambourin, carrots, a bow, a rainbow, cauliflowers

Page 7: a headset, a striped T-shirt

Page 8: a pearl necklace

Page 9: a tutu, a flamingo with an arabesque leg, a golden crown

Page 10: music scores, piano, a glass of water

Page 12: a bunch of flowers

Labyrinth

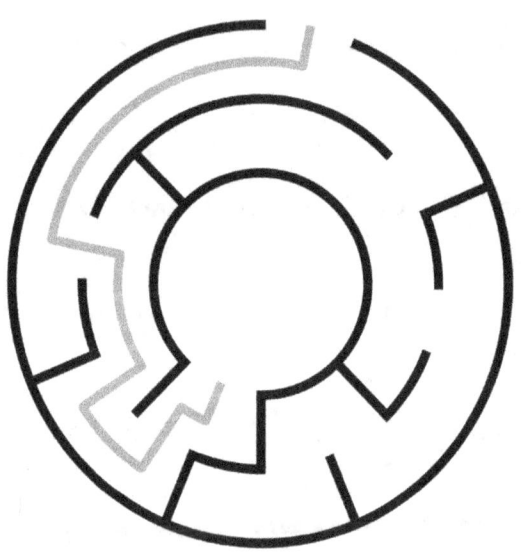

Here is your bookmark of the five ballet technical positions. Cut it out!

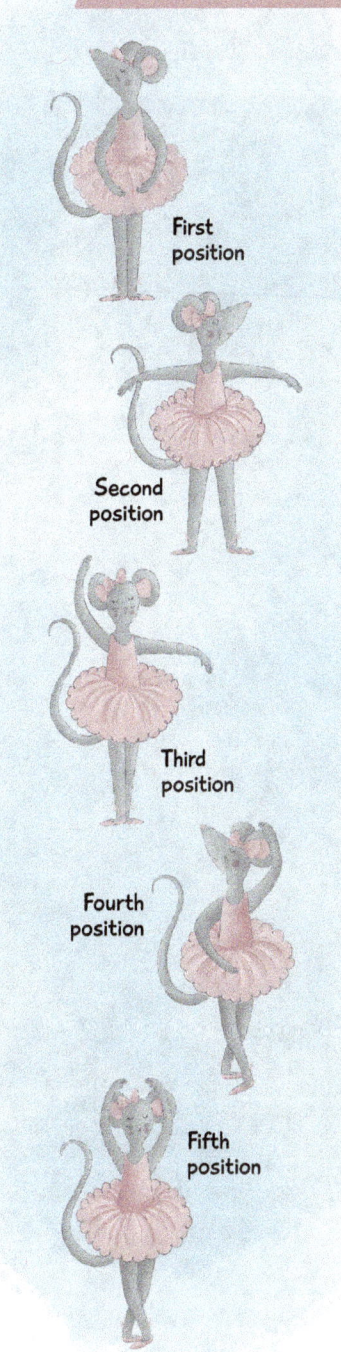

The 5 positions

First position

Second position

Third position

Fourth position

Fifth position

About the author

Former educator, professional dancer, dance teacher, and founder of her own Dance Academy, the author is proud to offer you her first activity book about dance and perseverance, dedicated to children aged from 4 to 7.

For a couple of years now, she has been willing to share some dance notions not only to the youngest, but also to their parents. In this first book, you will find dance activities to do at home, activities to practise memory, and activities to learn new specific vocabulary.

Mrs. Desrochers hopes that parents, dance teachers, and educators, looking for new activities, will enjoy this tool.

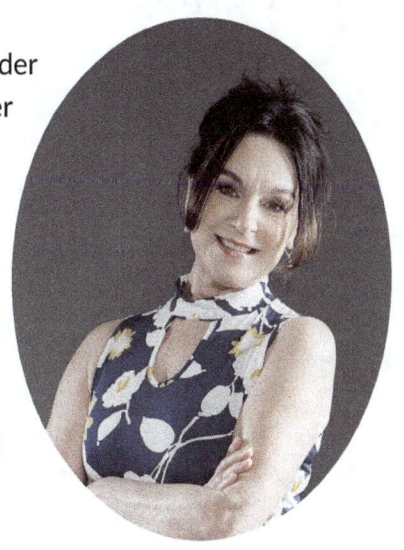

Photo credit: Annie Paquin

Follow us on the web

Instagram: www.instagram.com/academiedansebarbaradesrochers
Facebook: www.facebook.com/academiedansebarbara
YouTube: www.youtube.com/channel/UCnZphP3BTakDj7qAhMrbqmg
Website: www.ecolededansebarbara.com

Endnotes

1 Translator's note: Usually used in French during ballet classes. An English equivalent could be "cat's jump".
2 Translator's note: Usually used in French during ballet classes. An English equivalent could be "movement of the arms".
3 Translator's note: Usually used in French during ballet classes. An English equivalent could be "the group of dancers".
4 Translator's note: Usually used in French during ballet classes. An English equivalent could be "a spin".
5 Translator's note: Usually used in French during ballet classes. An English equivalent could be "whipped (turns)".
6 Translator's note: Usually used in French during ballet classes. An English equivalent could be "a Caper".
7 Translator's note: Usually used in French during ballet classes. An English equivalent could be "a ballet skirt".

www.ingramcontent.com/pod-product-compliance
Lightning Source LLC
Chambersburg PA
CBHW080352290526
45791CB00009BA/2845